Lean and Green Delights

Start to Feel Better With 50 Creative
and Delicious Recipes

Carmen Bellisario

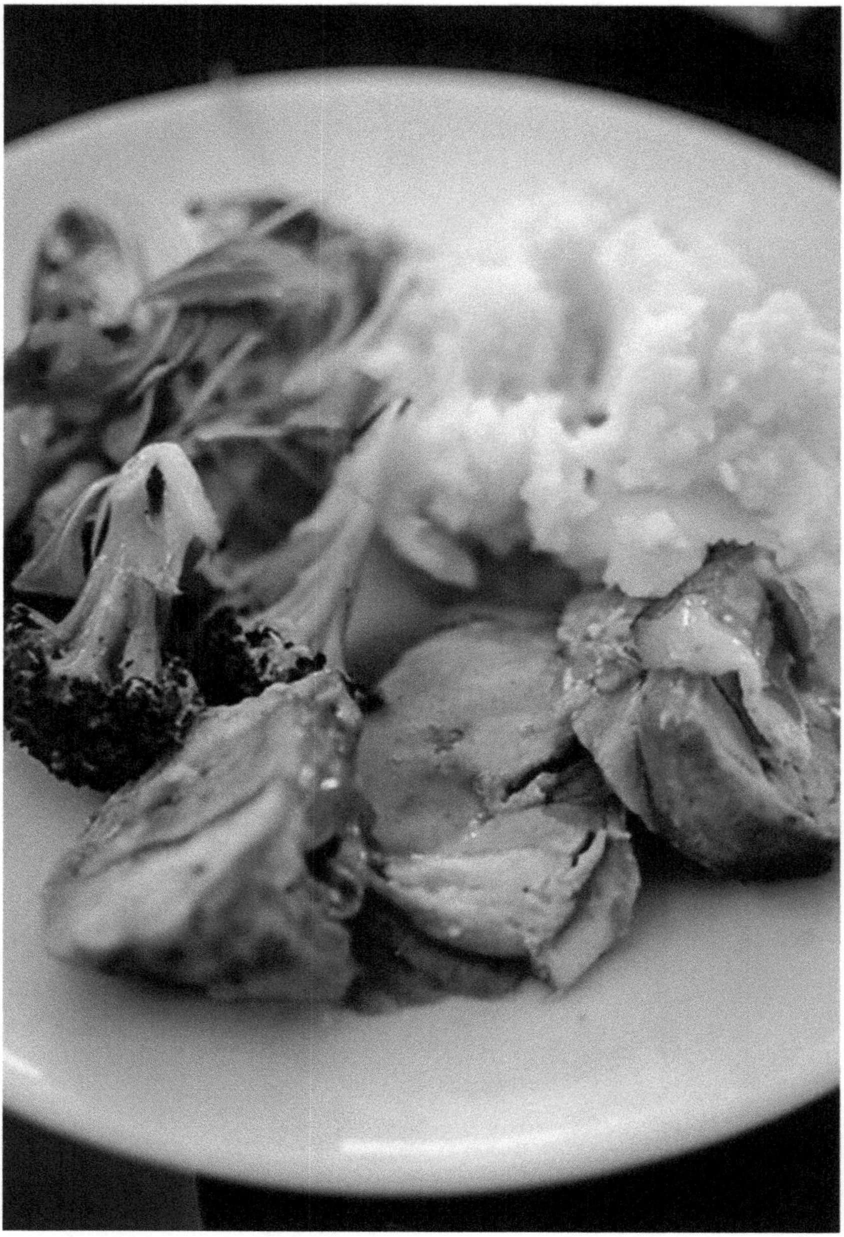

TABLE OF CONTENTS

Lightened-Up Bangers & Mash

Preparation time: 3 minutes

Cooking time: 20 minutes

Servings: 6

Ingredients:

- 6 (4-ounce) pork sausages (raw)
- 3 pounds of peeled and diced butternut squash
- 1 cup of chicken broth
- 1 chopped onion
- 1 tablespoon of Dijon mustard

Directions:

1. To prep, poke the sausages a couple of times.
2. Put squash in the pot and pour in the cup of chicken broth.
3. Stir in the Dijon.
4. Add steamer basket and pile in sausages with onion on top.
5. Seal the lid.
6. Hit "chicken/meat" and adjust time to 20 minutes.

7. When the time is up, hit "cancel" and quick-release.
8. Sausage should be cooked to 1450 F, while the squash is soft.
9. Serve!

Nutrition:

- Total calories: 506
- Protein: 19 g
- Carbs: 29 g
- Fat: 36 g
- Fiber: 5 g

Mexican-Braised Pork with Sweet Potatoes

Preparation time: 10 minutes

Cooking time: 25 minutes

Servings: 4

Ingredients:

- 3 pounds of pork loin
- 2 peeled and diced sweet potatoes
- 1 cup of tomato salsa
- ½ cup of chicken stock
- 1/3 cup of Mexican spice blend

Directions:

1. Season the pork all over with the spice blend.
2. Turn your cooker to "chicken/meat" and heat.
3. When hot, roast the pork on each side. If the meat sticks, pour in a little chicken broth.
4. When the pork is golden, pour in the salsa.

5. Tumble sweet potatoes on one side of the pot and seal the lid.
6. Adjust time to 25 minutes.
7. When the timer beeps, hit "cancel" and wait 10 minutes before quick-releasing.
8. The pork should be cooked to 1450 F, and the potatoes should be soft.
9. Remove the pork and rest 8-10 minutes before serving.

Nutrition:

- Total calories: 513
- Protein: 73 g
- Carbs: 17 g
- Fat: 14 g
- Fiber: 1 g

Apricot-Glazed Pork Chops

Preparation time: 15 minutes

Cooking time: 6 minutes

Servings: 6

Ingredients:

- 6 boneless pork chops
- ½ cup of apricot
- 1 tablespoon of balsamic vinegar
- 2 teaspoons of olive oil
- Black pepper to taste

Directions:

1. Add oil to your cooker and heat on "chicken/meat," leaving the lid off.
2. Sprinkle black pepper on the pork chops.
3. Roast chops in the cooker on each side till golden.
4. Mix balsamic and apricot preserving together.
5. Pour over the pork and seal the cooker lid.
6. Adjust cook time to 6 minutes.
7. When the time is up, hit "cancel" and quick-release.

8. Test temperature of pork—it should be 1450 F.

9. Allow to rest for 5 minutes before serving!

Nutrition:

- Total calories: 296
- Protein: 20 g
- Carbs: 18 g
- Fat: 16 g
- Fiber: 0

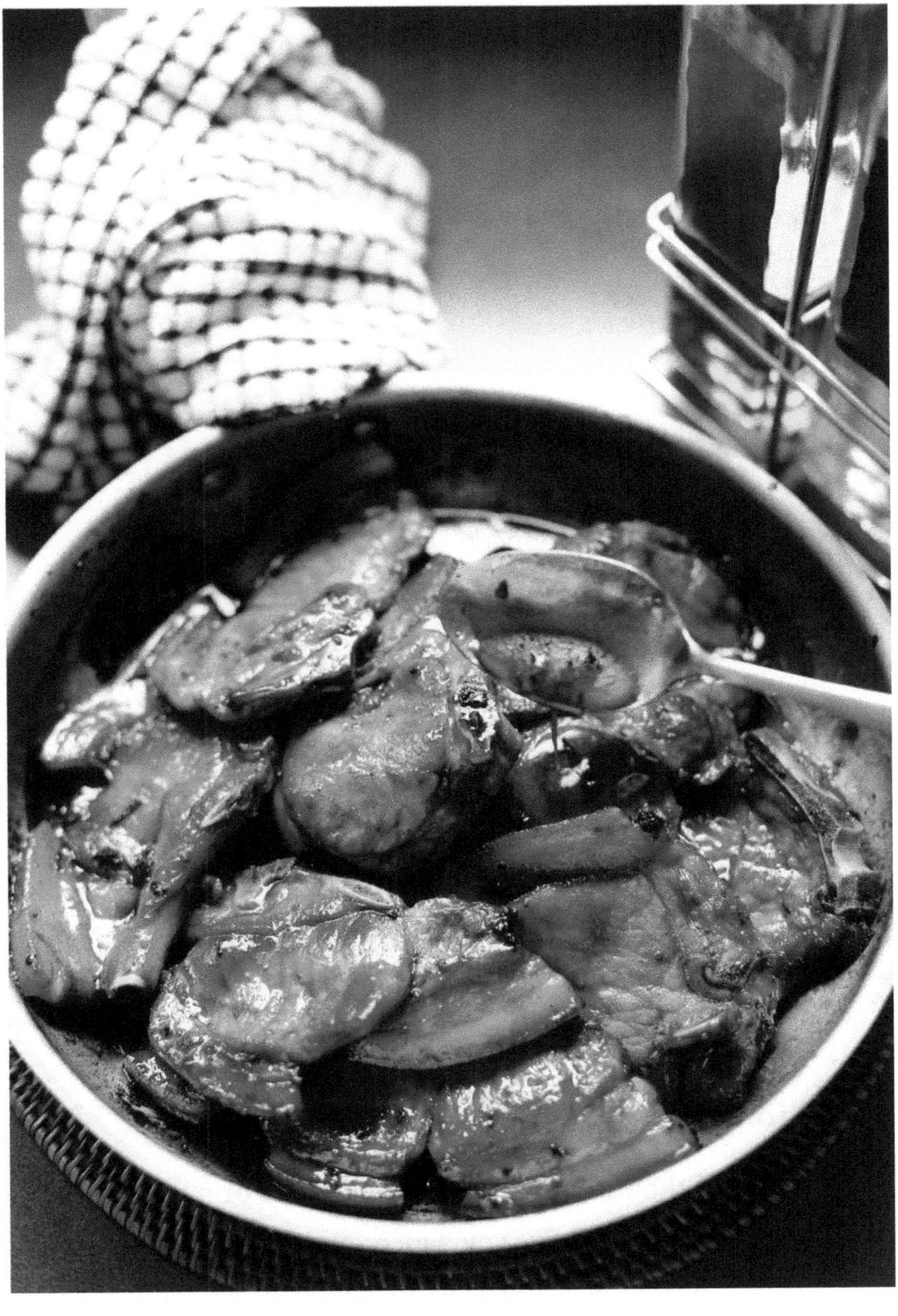

Simple Beef Stir-fry

Cooking time: 30 minutes

Servings: 4

Ingredients:

- 2 cups of vegetable stock
- 2 tablespoons of soy sauce
- 4 garlic cloves; chopped
- 2 teaspoons of chili powder
- 1 pound of top sirloin beef; thinly sliced
- 3 cups of broccoli; chopped into florets
- 1 cup of cremini mushrooms; sliced
- 1 cup of sugar snaps peas
- 4 green onions; sliced
- 1 tablespoon of fresh ginger; peeled and sliced
- 2 tablespoons of grapeseed oil

Directions:

1. Prepare the marinade in a shallow dish or a zip-lock bag, mix vegetable stock, soy sauce, and chili powder. If you desire more spices, add ½ teaspoon of cayenne pepper.

Toss the meat in the sauce and marinate for 10-15 minutes.

2. On high heat, add oil to the wok and when hot, put in ginger, broccoli, mushrooms, peas, green onions, and ¼ of the marinade, cook for about 3 minutes or until the broccoli softens. Add beef and the remaining marinade and cook until beef is browned. Serve hot.

Nutrition:

- Calories: 412
- Fat: 12 g
- Carbs: 14 g
- Protein: 24 g

Easy Pork Ribs

Preparation time: 10 minutes

Cooking time: 15 minutes

Servings: 6

Ingredients:

- 3 pounds of boneless pork ribs
- ½ cup of soy sauce
- ¼ cup of ketchup
- 2 tablespoons of olive oil
- Black pepper to taste

Directions:

1. Pour oil into your PPCXL and hit "chicken/meat," leaving the lid off.
2. When oil is hot, add ribs and roast till golden on each side.
3. In a bowl, mix black pepper, soy sauce, and ketchup.
4. Pour over ribs and seal the lid.
5. Adjust cook time to 15 minutes.

6. When the timer beeps, hit "cancel" and wait 5 minutes before quick-releasing.
7. Make sure pork is at least 1450 F before serving.

Nutrition:

- Total calories: 570
- Protein: 65 g
- Carbs: 0
- Fat: 27 g
- Fiber: 0

Sesame Beef and Vegetable Stir-fry

Preparation time: 5 minutes

Cooking time: 30 minutes

Servings: 4

Ingredients:

- 1 pound of lean top sirloin beef; cut into strips
- 1 bunch of asparagus; bottoms cut off and stalks halved
- 1 large handful of green beans; stemmed and cut in half
- 2 onions; diced
- 1 cup of vegetable stock
- 2 tablespoons of sesame seeds
- 3 teaspoons of basil
- 2 tablespoons of grape seed oil
- 2 cups of cooked brown rice

Directions:

1. On high heat, warm grapeseed oil in wok and cook beef until it turns brown. Remove from wok.

2. Put vegetable stock in the wok and heat until it's boiling. Add asparagus, green beans, and onions and cook until soft.
3. Add beef, sesame seeds, basil, and rice and cook until everything has absorbed the vegetable stock.
4. Serve warm and enjoy!

Nutrition:

- Calories: 234
- Fat: 5 g
- Carbs: 8 g
- Protein: 44 g

Roasted Lamb with Thyme and Garlic

Preparation time: 5 minutes

Cooking time: 30 minutes

Servings: 4

Ingredients:

- 3 pieces of lamb
- 3 cloves of garlic
- Olive oil
- Cooking spray
- Thyme
- Salt
- Pepper

Directions:

1. Season the meat on each side.
2. Pour a little vegetable oil spray.
3. Spread crushed garlic on each bit.
4. Preheat air fryer.

5. Put the meat into fryer and add thyme.

6. Wait till meat is fully cooked.

7. Serve.

Nutrition:

- Calories: 343
- Fat: 7 g
- Carbs: 6 g
- Protein: 34 g

Garlic-Cumin and Orange Juice Marinated Steak

Preparation time: 6 Minutes

Cooking time: 60 Minutes

Servings: 4

Ingredients:

- ¼ cup of orange juice
- 1 teaspoon of ground cumin
- 2 pounds of skirt steak; trimmed from excess fat
- 2 tablespoons of lime juice
- 2 tablespoons of olive oil
- 4 cloves of garlic; minced
- Salt and pepper to taste

Directions:

1. Place all the Ingredients in a bowl and allow to marinate in the fridge for at least 2 hours. Preheat the Cuisinart Air Fryer Oven to 390°F.
2. Place the grill pan accessory in the air fryer.

3. Grill for 15 minutes per batch and flip the meat every 8 minutes for even grilling.
4. Meanwhile, pour the marinade on a saucepan and allow to simmer for 10 minutes or until the sauce thickens.
5. Slice the meat and pour over the sauce.

Nutrition:

- Calories: 568
- Fat: 34.7 g
- Protein: 59.1 g
- Sugar: 1 g

Apple-Garlic Pork Loin

Preparation time: 5 minutes

Cooking time: 25 minutes

Servings: 12

Ingredients:

- One 3-pound of boneless pork loin roast
- One 12-ounce of jar of apple jelly
- 1/3 cup of water
- 1 tablespoon of Herbes de Provence
- 2 teaspoons of minced garlic

Directions:

1. Put cut of pork in your cooker. Cut in half if necessary.
2. Mix garlic, water, and jelly.
3. Pour over pork.
4. Season with Herbes de Provence.
5. Seal the lid.
6. Hit "chicken/meat" and adjust time to 25 minutes.
7. When the time is up, hit "cancel" and wait 10 minutes before quick-releasing.

8. Pork should be served at 1450 F. If not cooked through yet, hit "chicken/meat" and cook with the lid off until the temperature is reached.

9. Rest for 15 minutes before slicing.

Nutrition:

- Total calories: 236
- Protein: 26 g
- Carbs: 19 g
- Fat: 6 g
- Fiber: 0

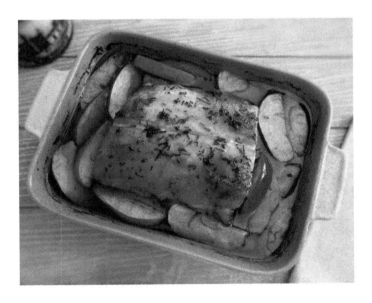

Peach-Mustard Pork Shoulder

Preparation time: 2 minutes

Cooking time: 55 minutes

Servings: 8

Ingredients:

- 4 pounds of pork shoulder
- 1 cup of peach
- 1 cup of white wine
- 1/3 cup of salt
- 1 tablespoon of grainy mustard

Directions:

1. Season the pork well with salt.
2. Mix mustard and peach, and rub on the pork.
3. Pour wine into cooker and add pork.
4. Seal the lid.
5. Hit "chicken/meat" and adjust time to 55 minutes.
6. When time is up, hit "cancel" and wait 10 minutes before quick-releasing.
7. Pork should be cooked to at least 1450 F.

8. Move pork to a plate and cover with foil for 15 minutes before slicing and serving.

Nutrition:

- Total calories: 583
- Protein: 44 g
- Carbs: 26 g
- Fat: 32 g
- Fiber: 0

Beef Taco Fried Egg Rolls

Preparation time: 10 Minutes

Cooking time: 12 Minutes

Servings: 8

Ingredients:

- 1 tsp. of cilantro
- 2 chopped garlic cloves
- 1 tbsp. of olive oil
- 1 cup of shredded Mexican cheese
- ½ packet of taco seasoning
- ½ can of cilantro lime rotel
- ½ chopped onion
- 16 egg roll wrappers
- 1-pound of lean ground beef

Directions:

1. Ensure that your Cuisinart Air Fryer Oven is preheated to 4000 F.

2. Add onions and garlic to a skillet, cooking till fragrant. Then add taco seasoning, pepper, salt, and beef, cooking till beef is broken up into tiny pieces and cooked thoroughly.
3. Add rotel and stir well.
4. Pour into the Oven rack/basket. Place the Rack on the middle-shelf of the Cuisinart Air Fryer Oven. Set temperature to 400°F, and set time to 8 minutes. Cook 8 minutes, flip, and cook another 4 minutes.
5. Served sprinkled with cilantro.

Nutrition:

- Calories: 348
- Fat: 11 g
- Protein: 24 g
- Sugar: 1 g

Beef with Beans

Preparation time: 10 Minutes

Cooking time: 13 Minutes

Servings: 4

Ingredients:

- 12 Oz. of Lean Steak
- 1 Onion; sliced
- 1 Can of Chopped Tomatoes
- 3/4 Cup of Beef Stock
- 4 tsps. of Fresh Thyme; chopped
- 1 Can of Red Kidney Beans
- Salt and Pepper to taste
- Oven Safe Bowl

Directions:

1. Preheat the Cuisinart Air Fryer Oven to 3900 F.
2. Set the temperature of the Fryer Oven to 390°F, and set time to 13 minutes, then Cook for 3 minutes. Add the meat and continue cooking for five minutes.

3. Add the tomatoes and their juice, beef broth, thyme and the beans and cook for a further 5 minutes. Season with black pepper to taste.

Nutrition:

- Calories: 178
- Fat: 14 g
- Protein: 9 g
- Fiber: 0 g

Lamb cacciatore

Preparation time: 5 minutes

Cooking time: 1 hour

Servings: 4

Ingredients:

- 4, 41 lb. of lamb; thighs and shoulders
- 2 tablespoons of flour
- 4 anchovies in salt
- 4 tablespoons of extra virgin olive oil
- 1 sprig of rosemary
- 4 cloves of garlic
- 1 glass of vinegar or white apple

Directions:

1. Cut lamb in regular slices with a thickness of about 2 cm.
2. Wash and dry the lamb pieces. Remove the needles from the rosemary twig, wash and dry them.
3. Peel the cloves of garlic, dig slices and put them in the jar of a food processor or a blender.

4. Mix the rosemary and chop everything. Put the mixture aside.

5. Pour the oil into a large pan, let it heat and roast the pieces of lamb over high heat. When the lamb is well browned, pepper and salts it.

6. Spread the chopped garlic and rosemary over the lamb and stir.

7. Cook covered for 30-45 minutes in the Air fryer, depending on the type of lamb and the thickness of the pieces, stirring occasionally and basting with a touch predicament if the sauce too dry.

8. Desiccate and desalted the anchovies and add the fillets to lamb at the top of cooking, stir and cook a couple of minutes to dissolve.

Nutrition:

- Calories: 209
- Fat: 4.3 g
- Carbs: 20 g
- Protein: 31 g

Beef Stroganoff

Preparation time: 10 Minutes

Cooking time: 14 Minutes

Servings: 4

Ingredients:

- 9 Oz. of soft Beef
- 1 Onion; chopped
- 1 tbsp. of Paprika
- 3/4 Cup of Sour Cream
- Salt and Pepper to taste
- Baking Dish

Directions:

1. Preheat the Cuisinart Air Fryer Oven to 3900 F.
2. Chop the meat and marinate it using paprika.
3. Add the chopped onions into the baking dish and heat for about 2 minutes in the Cuisinart Air Fryer Oven.
4. Add the meat into the dish when the onions are transparent, and cook for 5 minutes.

5. Once the meat is beginning to soften, pour in the soured cream and cook for an additional 7 minutes.
6. At this point, the liquid should have reduced. Season with salt and pepper and serve.

Nutrition:

- Calories: 254
- Fat: 21 g
- Protein: 33 g
- Fiber: 0 g

Lamb meat

Preparation time: 5 minutes

Cooking time: 30 minutes

Servings: 4

Ingredients:

- Mutton any lamb
- 3 tablespoons of oil
- Curcuma; according to desire
- Saffron; as desired
- Black pepper; as desired
- Salt; according to desire
- Cup water

Directions:

1. Preheat Air fryer to 392°F;
2. Cut the meat into small pieces.
3. Sprinkle the water over the meat and add turmeric, saffron, salt, and black pepper.
4. Leave the mixture into the fryer. Wait until the meat is fully cooked and red.

5. Serve with decorations (if needed).

Nutrition:

- Calories: 203
- Fat: 9 g
- Carbs: 25 g
- Protein: 43 g

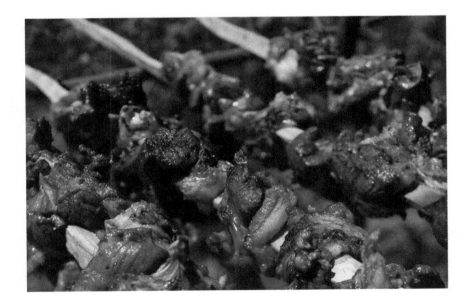

Lamb Fondue

Preparation time: 5

Cooking time: 30

Servings: 4

Ingredients:

- 1, 32 lb. of lamb fondue pieces
- 1 eggplant
- 1 zucchini
- 1 red pepper
- 1 liter of cooking oil skewers with a diced lamb and eggplant diced zucchini
- A square of red pepper

Directions:

1. Cut the vegetables into cubes of the same size as the fondue pieces.
2. Fit mini-skewers by changing the vegetables.
3. Cooking is done at the center of the table, with a fondue machine.

Nutrition:

- Calories: 140
- Fat: 0.3 g
- Carbs: 35 g
- Protein: 3 g

Laurel Lamb with Oregano

Preparation time: 5 minutes

Cooking time: 30 minutes

Servings: 4

Ingredients:

- 1, 65 lb. of lamb chops
- 3 cloves garlic
- 3 leaves laurel
- A sprig of oregano
- 2 tablespoons of chopped parsley
- 1 tablespoon of fresh or dried rosemary
- C / N virgin olive oil

Directions:

1. Put the chops on a platter and sprinkle with herbs and garlic, peeled and chopped. Add salt and pepper and marinate overnight.
2. The next day put the meat in a bowl and sprinkle with olive aciete. Leave to marinate at least 4 hours. Place beat a baking dish and shut either with transparent foil.

3. Preheat air fryer to 282°F for 1 minutes

4. Lower the temperature to 338°F and set to about 15 minutes.

5. Now remove meat from the Air fryer and raise the temperature of Air fryer to 428°F.

6. Remove the wrapping and return to the Air fryer for a couple of minutes or until the meat has a golden color.

7. Serve with roasted or fried potatoes.

Nutrition:

- Calories: 206
- Fat: 21.3 g
- Carbs: 15 g
- Protein: 13 g

Airfried lamb with potatoes

Preparation time: 5 minutes

Cooking time: 2 hours and 30 minutes

Servings: 4

Ingredients:

- Rack of lamb
- Potatoes
- White wine
- Vegetables soup
- Garlic teeth
- Branches rosemary
- Grain Pepper
- Coarse salt

Directions:

1. Preheat the Air fryer to 392°F.
2. Place the rib in a suitable baking dish, sprinkle with coarse salt and peppercorns, then add whole garlic teeth and branches of rosemary, add oil and a few wine.
3. Put in the Air fryer and lower the temperature to 347°F.

4. Prepare a vegetable stock which can be added when it dries.

5. At that temperature, cook the rib for 2 hours. After the first hour, close up and add the potatoes, then you are ready to start serving.

Nutrition:

- Calories: 231
- Fat: 11 g
- Carbs: 12 g
- Protein: 25 g

Braised & Baked Lamb Stew

Preparation time: 5 minutes

Cooking time: 30 minutes

Servings: 4

Ingredients:

- 1 unit of lamb shoulder (1, 54 lb.)
- 1 piece of green pepper
- 1 clove of onion
- 1 clove of tomato
- 4 garlic cloves
- 0, 77 lb. of potato
- 1 pinch of pepper and salt
- 1 bay leaf
- ½ teaspoon of oregano
- 1 cup of white wine
- ½ cup of broth
- Meat

Directions:

1. Prepare all the Ingredients. Cut lamb shoulder into two parts. Cover potatoes slightly. In a special baking pan, place in layers the pepper, tomato, onion and garlic.
2. Season with all the seasonings, wine and broth.
3. Place the lamb pieces on all the vegetables and bring to a preheated Air fryer at 356°F for 90 minutes.
4. During the frying process, check the lamb every 20-30 minutes, and turn it.
5. 15 minutes to end of cooking, open the Air fryer and place the potatoes in the pan.
6. When you finish cooking, potatoes should be softer.

Nutrition:

- Calories: 1123
- Fat: 5 g
- Carbs: 20 g
- Protein: 31 g

Lamb Meatballs with Feta

Preparation time: 5 minutes

Cooking time: 30 minutes

Servings: 4

Ingredients:

- 0, 33 lb. of lamb minces
- 1 slice of stale white bread; turned into fine crumbs
- 0, 11 lb. of Greek feta; crumbled
- 1 tablespoon of fresh oregano; finely chopped
- ½ tablespoon of grated lemon peel
- Freshly ground black pepper

Directions:

1. Preheat the Air Fryer to 392°F.
2. Mix the mince in a bowl with the bread crumbs, feta, oregano, lemon rind, and black pepper, thoroughly kneading everything together.
3. Cut the mixture in 10 equal portions to form round balls.
4. Place this dish in the basket inside the oven dish. Slide the basket into the Air Fryer. Set the timer to 8 minutes

and bake the mince balls until they are nicely brown and done.

5. Serve the meatballs hot in a platter with tapas forks.

Nutrition:

- Calories: 300
- Fat: 2.5 g
- Carbs: 5 g
- Protein: 13 g

Garlic Lamb with Rosemary

Preparation time: 5 minutes

Cooking time: 45 minutes

Servings: 4

Ingredients:

- 1 leg of lamb
- Branches of fresh rosemary
- Several garlic cloves
- 5 pepper (or otherwise black pepper)
- Fleur de sel
- 2 onions
- 2, 2 lb. of potatoes
- Extra virgin olive oil

Directions:

1. Preheat the Air fryer to 356°F.
2. Remove the blade bone of the lamb. Remove excess fat.
3. Dry the piece of blood residues. If you removed the bone, add salt, and pepper inside, then close and tie round with

kitchen string. Peel the garlic cloves and cut 3 pieces lengthwise. Wash the rosemary.

4. Add garlic and rosemary all over the outer surface of the lamb leg. To do this, make a deep incision with a knife and put inside a bit of garlic and a sprig of rosemary. Coat the surface generously with sea salt and 5 peppers.

5. Peel the potatoes, rinse, and cut thick slices of 5 mm thickness. Peel onions and cut them into thick equal slices.

6. Grease the bottom of the baking tray with olive oil. Place the potato slices on the tray and spread the onion on top.

7. Place the lamb with garlic and rosemary in the center and sprinkle with olive oil.

8. Bake each 1 lb. of meat at medium heat for 15 minutes so that it is a little done and 20 to 25 minutes per 1, 1 lb to the point that it is either done.

9. A half cooking, add half glass of water to the potato or a little more, as needed.

10. If the surface is browning too quickly, cover with baking paper. Optionally, 15 minutes before the end of cooking, sprinkle top with melted butter and finish uncovered.

Nutrition:

- Calories: 365
- Fat: 21 g
- Carbs: 11 g

- Protein: 15 g

Roasted Lamb with Honey

Preparation time: 5 minutes

Cooking time: 30 minutes

Servings: 4

Ingredients:

- 1, 32 lb. of lamb
- 2 tablespoons of mustard tarragon
- 2 tablespoons of rosemary honey
- 2 tablespoons of soy
- 1 teaspoon of rosemary; chopped
- 2 cloves of garlic; minced
- C / N Extra virgin olive
- 0, 88 lb of potatoes; peeled and chopped
- Salt and black pepper

Directions:

1. Put the meat to macerate the night before with mustard, honey, soy, chopped rosemary, garlic, 1 chorretón oil, salt and pepper.
2. Cook the potatoes and put aside.
3. Place meat in a preheated Air fryer at 392°F for 20 minutes. Remove and add the potatoes.
4. Return meat to Air fryer and lower the temperature to 338°F. When the meat is cooked, remove and serve with potatoes.

Nutrition:

- Calories: 243
- Fat: 22 g
- Carbs: 13 g
- Protein: 20 g

Baked Patties

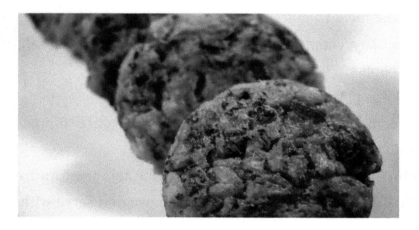

Preparation time: 10 minutes

Cooking time: 15 minutes

Servings: 4

Ingredients:

- 1 lb. of ground lamb
- 1 teaspoon of ground coriander
- 1 teaspoon of ground cumin
- ¼ cup of fresh parsley; chopped
- ¼ cup of onion; minced
- ¼ teaspoon of cayenne pepper
- ½ teaspoon of ground allspice
- 1 teaspoon of ground cinnamon
- 1 tablespoon of garlic; minced

- ¼ teaspoon of pepper
- 1 teaspoon of kosher salt

Directions:

1. Preheat the oven to 4500 F.
2. Add all the Ingredients into a big bowl and blend until well mixed.
3. Make small meatballs from meat mixture and place on a baking tray and lightly flatten the meatballs with the back of a spoon.
4. Bake in preheated oven for 12-15 minutes.
5. Serve and enjoy.

Nutrition:

- Calories: 112
- Fat: 4.3 g
- Carbohydrates: 1.3 g
- Sugar: 0.2 g
- Protein: 16 g
- Cholesterol: 51 mg

Lamb tagine

Servings: 4

Ingredients:

- 1.32 lb. of lamb shoulder
  - oz. of white wine
- 0.088 lb. of pitted black olives
- 04 ml of water
- 0.033 lb. of fresh ginger
- 0.015 lb. of lemon zest
- 1 spoon of garlic powder
- 1 spoon of oil
- 1 spoon of parsley
- 1 spoon of coriander
- 1 dose of saffron
- 1 spoon of maizena
- Salt
- Pepper

Directions:

1. Slice the lamb into cubes of 3-4 cm and coat the pieces of Maizena. Chop the ginger.
2. In a bowl, mix the wine and water.
3. Grate the lemon
4. Put the olives, ginger, lemon peel, parsley, coriander, saffron, and garlic in air fryer—handle side of tank.
5. Arrange the lamb in the bowl opposite the handle. Pour the mixture over the spices. Spread the oil over the lamb. Close the hood.
6. Start cooking.

Nutrition:

- Calories: 105
- Fat: 29 g
- Carbs: 2 g
- Protein: 23 g

Lamb chops

Preparation time: 10 minutes

Cooking time: 25 minutes

Servings: 4

Ingredients:

- Oregano
- Thyme
- Garlic
- Salt
- Pepper

Directions:

1. Cut the vegetables into cubes of the same size of fondue pieces.
2. Fit mini-skewers by changing the vegetables.
3. Cooking is completed at the middle of the table, with a fondue machine.

Nutrition:

- Calories: 279
- Fat: 11 g
- Carbs: 13 g
- Protein: 43 g

Breaded and crispy lamb chops

Preparation time: 5 minutes

Cooking time: 30 minutes

Servings: 4

Ingredients:

- 2 eggs
- 8 lean lamb chops
- 0.044 lb. of flour
- 0.44 lb. of breadcrumbs (made of crumbled breadcrumbs)
- 52.79 oz. of cooking oil

Directions:

1. Beat the eggs with salt and pepper.
2. Pass the lamb chops, first in the flour, and then in the eggs, and eventually in the bread crumbs. To get a thicker crust, pass the chops again in the eggs and then in the bread crumbs.
3. Heat the oil in the air fryer at approx. 338°F.
4. Fry the chops until they're golden brown.

5. Allow them drain on paper towels, sprinkle with salt and pepper to taste and store (uncovered) in an oven.

Nutrition:

- Calories: 142
- Fat: 9.3 g
- Carbs: 5 g
- Protein: 53 g

Beef Patties

Preparation time: 10 minutes

Cooking time: 8 minutes

Servings: 5

Ingredients:

- 1 lb. of ground beef
- 1 egg; lightly beaten
- 3 tablespoon of almond flour
- 1 small onion; grated
- 2 tablespoon of fresh parsley; chopped
- 1 teaspoon of dry oregano
- 1 teaspoon of dry mint
- Pepper
- Salt

Directions:

1. Using a sharp knife, make small cuts all over the meat then insert garlic slivers into the cuts.

2. In a small bowl, mix together marjoram, thyme, oregano, pepper, salt, and rub all over the roast lamb.

3. Place roast lamb into the slow cooker.

4. Cover and cook on low for 8 hours.

5. Serve and enjoy.

Nutrition:

- Calories: 188
- Fat: 6.6 g
- Carbohydrates: 1.7 g
- Sugar: 0.7 g
- Protein: 28.9 g
- Cholesterol: 114 mg

Tender & Juicy Lamb Roast

Preparation time: 10 minutes

Cooking time: 8 hours

Servings: 8

Ingredients:

- 4 lbs. of lamb roast; boneless
- ½ teaspoon of thyme
- 1 teaspoon of oregano
- 4 garlic cloves; cut into slivers
- ½ teaspoon of marjoram
- ¼ teaspoon of pepper
- 2 teaspoons of salt

Directions:

1. Using a sharp knife, make small cuts all over meat then insert garlic slivers into the cuts.
2. In a small bowl, mix together the marjoram, thyme, oregano, pepper, salt, and rub all over lamb roast.
3. Place lamb roast into the slow cooker.
4. Cover and cook on low for 8 hours.

5. Serve and enjoy.

Nutrition:

- Calories: 605
- Fat: 48 g
- Carbohydrates: 0.7 g
- Sugar: 1 g
- Protein: 36 g
- Cholesterol: 160 mg

Basil Cheese Pork Roast

Preparation time: 10 minutes

Cooking time: 6 hours

Servings: 8

Ingredients:

- 2 lbs. of lean pork roast, boneless
- 1 teaspoon of garlic powder
- 1 tablespoon of parsley
- ½ cup of cheddar cheese; grated
- 30 oz. of can tomatoes; diced
- 1 teaspoon of dried oregano
- 1 teaspoon of dried basil
- Pepper
- Salt

Directions:

1. Add the meat into the crock pot.
2. Mix together tomatoes, oregano, basil, garlic powder, parsley, cheese, pepper, salt, and pour over the meat.

3. Cover and cook on low for 6 hours.

4. Serve and enjoy.

Nutrition:

- Calories: 260
- Fat: 9 g
- Carbohydrates: 5.5 g
- Sugar: 3.5 g
- Protein: 35 g
- Cholesterol: 97 mg

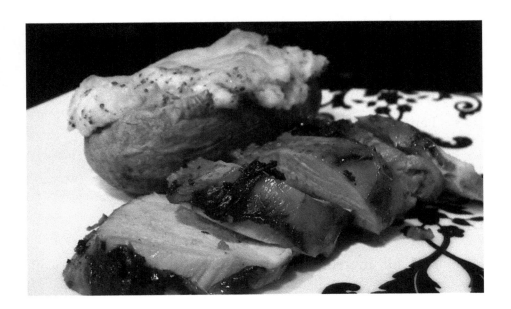

Feta Lamb Patties

Preparation time: 10 minutes

Cooking time: 12 minutes

Servings: 4

Ingredients:

- 1 lb. of ground lamb
- 1/2 teaspoon of garlic powder
- 1/2 cup of feta cheese; crumbled
- 1/4 cup of mint leaves; chopped
- 1/4 cup of roasted red pepper; chopped
- 1/4 cup of onion; chopped
- Pepper
- Salt

Directions:

1. Add all Ingredients into a bowl and blend until well mixed.
2. Spray pan with cooking spray and heat over medium-high heat.

3. Make small patties from meat mixture and place on hot pan and cook for 6-7 minutes on all sides.

4. Serve and enjoy.

Nutrition:

- Calories: 270
- Fat: 12 g
- Carbohydrates: 2.9 g
- Sugar: 1.7 g
- Protein: 34.9 g
- Cholesterol: 119 mg

Cheesy Ground Beef and Mac Taco Casserole

Preparation time: 10 Minutes

Cooking time: 25 Minutes

Servings: 5

Ingredients:

- 1-ounce of shredded Cheddar cheese
- 1-ounce of shredded Monterey Jack cheese
- 2 tablespoons of chopped green onions
- 1/2 (10.75 ounce) can of condensed tomato soup
- 1/2-pound of lean ground beef
- 1/2 cup of crushed tortilla chips
- 1/4-pound of macaroni; cooked according to manufacturer's
- 1/4 cup of chopped onion
- 1/4 cup of sour cream (optional)
- 1/2 (1.25 ounce) package of taco seasoning mix
- 1/2 (14.5 ounce) can of diced tomatoes

Directions:

1. Lightly grease baking pan of air fryer with cooking spray. Add onion and ground beef. Cook on 360°F for 10 minutes. Halfway into Cooking time, stir and crumble ground beef.
2. Add taco seasoning, diced tomatoes, and tomato soup. Mix well in pasta.
3. Sprinkle crushed tortilla chips. Sprinkle cheese.
4. Cook for 15 minutes at 390°F or until tops are lightly browned and cheese is melted.
5. Serve and enjoy.

Nutrition:

- Calories: 329
- Fat: 17 g
- Protein: 15.6 g

Beefy Steak Topped with Chimichurri Sauce

Preparation time: 5 Minutes

Cooking time: 60 Minutes

Servings: 6

Ingredients:

- 1 cup of commercial chimichurri
- 3 pounds of steak
- Salt and pepper to taste

Directions:

1. Place all Ingredients in a Ziploc bag and marinate in the fridge for 2 hours.
2. Preheat the air fryer to 390°F.
3. Place the grill pan accessory in the air fryer.
4. Grill the skirt steak for 20 minutes per batch.
5. Flip the steak every 10 minutes for even grilling.

Nutrition:

- Calories: 507
- Fat: 27 g
- Protein: 63 g

Mozzarella Sticks

Preparation time: 8 minutes

Cooking time: 2 minutes

Servings: 2

Ingredients:

- 1 large whole egg
- 3 sticks of mozzarella cheese in half (frozen overnight)
- 2 tablespoon of grated parmesan cheese
- 1/2 cup of almond flour
- 1/4 cup of coconut oil
- 2 1/2 teaspoons of Italian seasoning blend
- 1 tablespoon of chopped parsley
- 1/2 teaspoon of salt

Directions:

1. Heat the coconut oil in a medium sizeed cast-iron skillet over low-medium heat.
2. In the meantime, crack the egg in a small bowl and beat it well.

3. Take another bowl of medium size and add parmesan cheese, almond flour, and seasonings to it. Whisk the Ingredients together until a smooth mixture is available.

4. Take the overnight frozen mozzarella stick and dip it in the beaten egg, then coat it well with the dry mixture. Do the same with all the remaining cheese sticks.

5. Place all the coated sticks in the preheated skillet and cook them for 2 minutes or until they start having a golden brown look on all sides.

6. Remove from the skillet once cooked properly and place over a towel so that any extra oil gets absorbed.

7. Sprinkle parsley over the sticks if you desire and serve with keto marinara sauce.

Nutrition:

- Calories: 430 g
- Fat: 39 g
- Carbohydrates: 10 g
- Protein: 20 g

Sausage and Cheese Dip

Preparation time: 10 minutes

Cooking time: 130 minutes

Servings: 28

Ingredients:

- 8 ounces cream cheese
- A pinch of salt and black pepper
- 16 ounces of sour cream
- 8 ounces of pepper jack cheese; chopped
- 15 ounces of canned tomatoes mixed with habaneros
- 1-pound of Italian sausage; ground
- ¼ cup of green onions; chopped

Directions:

1. Heat up a pan over medium heat, add sausage, stir and cook until it browns.
2. Add tomatoes mix, stir and cook for 4 minutes more.
3. Add a pinch of salt, black pepper, and the green onions, stir and cook for 4 minutes.

4. Spread pepper jack cheese on the bottom of your slow cooker.
5. Add cream cheese, sausage mix, and soured cream, cover and cook on High for 2 hours.
6. Uncover your slow cooker, stir dip, transfer to a bowl, and serve.
7. Enjoy!

Nutrition:

- Calories: 132
- Protein: 6.79 g
- Fat: 9.58 g
- Carbohydrates: 6.22 g
- Sodium: 362 mg

Stuffed Avocado

Preparation time: 10 minutes

Cooking time: 0 minute

Servings: 2

Ingredients:

- 1 avocado; halved and pitted
- 10 ounces of canned tuna; drained
- 2 tablespoons of sun-dried tomatoes; chopped
- 1 and ½ tablespoon of basil pesto
- 2 tablespoons of black olives; pitted and chopped
- Salt and black pepper to the taste
- 2 teaspoons of pine nuts; toasted and chopped
- 1 tablespoon of basil; chopped

Directions:

1. In a bowl, mix the tuna with the sun-dried tomatoes and the rest of the Ingredients except the avocado and stir.
2. Stuff the avocado halves with the tuna mix and serve as an appetizer.

Nutrition:

- Calories: 233
- Fat: 9 g
- Fiber: 3.5 g
- Carbs: 11.4 g
- Protein: 5.6 g

Tasty Onion and Cauliflower Dip

Preparation time: 20 minutes

Cooking time: 30 minutes

Servings: 24

Ingredients:

- 1 ½ cups of chicken stock
- 1 cauliflower head; florets separated
- ¼ cup of mayonnaise
- ½ cup of yellow onion; chopped
- ¾ cup of cream cheese
- ½ teaspoon of chili powder
- ½ teaspoon of cumin; ground
- ½ teaspoon of garlic powder
- Salt and black pepper to the taste

Directions:

1. Put the stock in a pot, add cauliflower and onion, heat up over medium heat, and cook for 30 minutes.

2. Add chili powder, salt, pepper, cumin, garlic powder, and stir.
3. Also, add cheese and stir a touch until it melts.
4. Blend using an immersion blender and blend with the mayo.
5. Transfer to a bowl and keep in the fridge for 2 hours before you serve it.
6. Enjoy!

Nutrition:

- Calories: 40
- Protein: 1.23 g
- Fat: 3.31 g
- Carbohydrates: 1.66 g
- Sodium: 72 mg

Avocado Taco Boats

Preparation time: 5 minutes

Cooking time: 20 minutes

Servings: 4

Ingredients:

- 4 grape tomatoes
- 2 large avocados
- 1 lb. of ground beef
- 4 tablespoon of taco seasoning
- 3/4 cup of shredded sharp cheddar cheese
- 4 slices of pickled jalapeño
- 1/4 cup of salsa
- 3 shredded romaine leaves
- 1/4 cup of sour cream
- 2/3 cup of water

Directions:

1. Take a skillet of huge size, grease it with oil, and warmth it over medium-high heat. Cook the bottom beef in it for 10-15 minutes or until it has a brownish look.
2. Once the meat browns, drain the grease from the skillet and add the water and the taco seasoning.
3. Reduce the heat once the taco seasoning gets mixed well and simmer for 8-10 minutes.
4. Take both avocados and cut in halves using a sharp knife.
5. Take each avocado shell and fill it with ¼ of the shredded romaine leaves.
6. Fill each shell with ¼ of the cooked ground beef.
7. Do the topping with soured cream, cheese, jalapeno, salsa, and tomato before you serve the delicious avocado taco.

Nutrition:

- Calories: 430
- Fat: 35 g
- Carbohydrates: 5 g
- Protein: 32 g

Pesto Crackers

Preparation time: 10 minutes

Cooking time: 17 minutes

Servings: 6

Ingredients:

- ½ teaspoon of baking powder
- Salt and black pepper to the taste
- 1 and ¼ cups of almond flour
- ¼ teaspoon of basil; dried
- 1 garlic clove; minced
- 2 tablespoons of basil pesto
- A pinch of cayenne pepper
- 3 tablespoons of ghee

Directions:

1. In a bowl, mix salt, pepper, baking powder, and almond flour.
2. Add garlic, cayenne, and basil and stir.
3. Add pesto and whisk.
4. Also, add ghee and blend your dough with your finger.

5. Spread this dough on a lined baking sheet, then put in the oven at 3250 F and bake for 17 minutes.
6. Set aside to cool, then cut your crackers and serve them as a snack.
7. Enjoy!

Nutrition:

- Calories: 9
- Protein: 0.41 g
- Fat: 0.14 g
- Carbohydrates: 1.86 g
- Sodium: 2 mg

Chicken and Mushrooms

Preparation time: 10 minutes

Cooking time: 15 minutes

Servings: 6

Ingredients:

- 2 chicken breasts
- 1 cup of sliced white champignons
- 1 cup of sliced green chilies
- 1/2 cup of scallions; hacked
- 1 teaspoon of chopped garlic
- 1 cup of low-fat cheddar shredded cheese (1-1.5 lb. grams fat / ounce)
- 1 tablespoon of olive oil
- 1 tablespoon of butter

Directions:

1. Fry the chicken breasts with olive oil.
2. Add salt and pepper as needed.
3. Grill breasts of chicken in a plate with grill.

4. For every serving, weigh 4 ounces of chicken. (Make two Servings, save leftovers for an additional meal).
5. In a butter pan, stir in mushrooms, green peppers, scallions, and garlic until smooth, and a bit dark.
6. Place the chicken in a baking platter.
7. Cover with mushroom combination.
8. Top with ham.
9. Place the cheese in a 3500 F oven until it melts.

Nutrition:

- Carbohydrates: 2 g
- Protein: 23 g
- Fat: 11 g
- Cholesterol: 112 mg
- Sodium: 198 mg
- Potassium: 261 mg

Marinated Eggs

Preparation time: 2 hours and 10 minutes

Cooking time: 7 minutes

Servings: 4

Ingredients:

- 6 eggs
- 1 and ¼ cups of water
- ¼ cup of unsweetened rice vinegar
- 2 tablespoons of coconut aminos
- Salt and black pepper to the taste
- 2 garlic cloves; minced
- 1 teaspoon of stevia
- 4 ounces of cream cheese
- 1 tablespoon of chives; chopped

Directions:

1. Put the eggs in a pot, add water to cover, bring to a boil over medium heat, cover and cook for 7 minutes.

2. Rinse eggs with cold water and set them aside to chill down.
3. In a bowl, mix one cup of water with coconut aminos, vinegar, stevia, garlic, and whisk well.
4. Put the eggs in this mix, cover with a kitchen towel, and put them aside for 2 hours, turning from time to time.
5. Peel eggs, cut in halves, and put egg yolks in a bowl.
6. Add ¼ cup water, cream cheese, salt, pepper, chives, and stir well.
7. Stuff egg whites with this mix and serve them.
8. Enjoy!

Nutrition:

- Calories: 289
- Protein: 15.86 g
- Fat: 22.62 g
- Carbohydrates: 4.52 g
- Sodium: 288 mg

Lamb Stuffed Avocado

Preparation time: 10 minutes

Cooking time: 40 minutes

Servings: 4

Ingredients:

- 2 avocados
- 1 1/2 cup of minced lamb
- 1/2 cup of cheddar cheese; grated
- 1/2 cup of parmesan cheese; grated
- 2 tbsps. of almond; chopped
- 1 tbsp. of coriander; chopped
- 2 tbsps. of olive oil
- 1 tomato; chopped
- 1 jalapeno; chopped
- Salt and pepper to taste
- 1 tsp. of garlic, chopped
- 1-inch ginger; chopped

Directions:

1. Cut the avocados in half. Remove the pit and scoop out some flesh so as to be able to stuff it later.
2. In a skillet, add half the oil.
3. Toss the ginger, garlic for 1 minute.
4. Add the lamb and toss for 3 minutes.
5. Add the tomato, coriander, parmesan, jalapeno, salt, pepper, and cook for 2 minutes.
6. Take off the heat. Stuff the avocados.
7. Sprinkle the almonds, cheddar cheese, and add olive oil on top.
8. Add to a baking sheet and bake for 30 minutes. Serve.

Nutrition:

- Fat: 19.5 g
- Cholesterol: 167.5 mg
- Sodium: 410.7 mg
- Potassium: 617.1 mg
- Carbohydrate: 13.1 g

Chili Mango and Watermelon Salsa

Preparation time: 5 minutes

Cooking time: 0 minutes

Servings: 12

Ingredients:

- 1 red tomato; chopped
- Salt and black pepper to the taste
- 1 cup of watermelon; seedless, peeled and cubed
- 1 red onion; chopped
- 2 mangos; peeled and chopped
- 2 chili peppers; chopped
- ¼ cup of cilantro; chopped
- 3 tablespoons of lime juice
- Pita chips for serving

Directions:

1. In a bowl, mix the tomato with the watermelon, the onion, and the rest of the Ingredients except the pita chips, and toss well.
2. Divide the mix into small cups and serve with pita chips on the side.

Nutrition:

- Calories: 62
- Fat: 4 g
- Fiber: 1.3 g
- Carbs: 3.9 g
- Protein: 2.3 g

Pumpkin Muffins

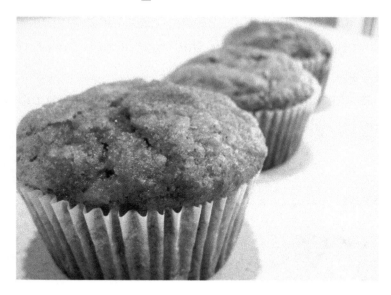

Preparation time: 10 minutes

Cooking time: 15 minutes

Servings: 18

Ingredients:

- ¼ cup of sunflower seed butter
- ¾ cup of pumpkin puree
- 2 tablespoons of flaxseed meal
- ¼ cup of coconut flour
- ½ cup of erythritol
- ½ teaspoon of nutmeg; ground

- 1 teaspoon of cinnamon; ground
- ½ teaspoon of baking soda
- 1 egg ½ teaspoon of baking powder
- A pinch of salt

Directions:

1. In a bowl, mix butter with pumpkin puree and egg and blend well.
2. Add flaxseed meal, coconut flour, erythritol, baking soda, baking powder, nutmeg, cinnamon, a pinch of salt, and stir well.
3. Spoon this into a greased muffin pan, put in the oven at 3500 F and bake for 15 minutes.
4. Leave muffins to chill down and serve them as a snack.
5. Enjoy!

Nutrition:

- Calories: 65
- Protein: 2.82 g
- Fat: 5.42 g
- Carbohydrates: 2.27 g
- Sodium: 57 mg

Chicken Enchilada Bake

Preparation time: 20 minutes

Cooking time: 50 minutes

Servings: 5

Ingredients:

- 5 oz. of Shredded chicken breast (boil and shred ahead) or 99 percent fat-free white chicken can be used in a pan.
- 1 can of tomato paste
- 1 low sodium chicken broth can be fat-free
- 1/4 cup of cheese with low fat mozzarella
- 1 tablespoon of oil
- 1 tbsp. of salt
- Ground cumin, chili powder, garlic powder, oregano, and onion powder (all to taste)
- 1 to 2 zucchinis sliced vertically (similar to lasagna noodles) into thin lines
- Sliced (optional) olives

Directions:

1. Add vegetable oil in sauce pan over medium-high heat, stir in Ingredients and seasonings, and heat in chicken stock for 2-3 min.
2. Turn heat to low for 15 min, stirring regularly to boil.
3. Set aside and cool to ambient temperature.
4. Pull-strip of zucchini through enchilada sauce and lay flat on the pan's bottom in a small baking pan.
5. Next, add the chicken with the 1/4 cup of enchilada sauce and blend it.
6. Place chicken to the end to end duvet of the baking tray.
7. Sprinkle some bacon over the chicken.
8. Add another layer of the pulled zucchini via enchilada sauce (similar to lasagna making).
9. When needed, cover with the remaining cheese and olives on top. Bake for 35 to 40 minutes.
10. Keep an eye on them.
11. When the cheese starts getting golden, cover with foil.
12. Serve and enjoy!

Nutrition:

- Calories: 312
- Carbohydrates: 21.3 g
- Protein: 27 g

- Fat: 10.2 g

Greek Tuna Salad Bites

Preparation time: 5 Minutes

Cooking time: 10 Minutes

Servings: 6

Ingredients:

- Cucumbers (2 medium)
- White tuna (2 - 6 oz. cans)
- Lemon juice (half of 1 lemon)
- Red bell pepper (.5 cup)
- Sweet/red onion (.25 cup)
- Black olives (.25 cup)
- Garlic (2 tablespoons)
- Olive oil (2 tablespoons)
- Fresh parsley (2 tablespoons)
- Dried oregano
- salt & pepper (as desired)

Directions:

1. Drain and flake the tuna. Juice the lemon. Dice/chop the onions, olives, pepper, parsley, and garlic. Slice each of the cucumbers into thick rounds (skin off or on).
2. In a mixing container, mix the rest of the Ingredients.
3. Place a heaping spoonful of salad onto the rounds and enjoy.

Nutrition:

- Calories: 400
- Fats: 22 g
- Carbs: 26 g
- Fiber Content: 8 g
- Protein: 30 g

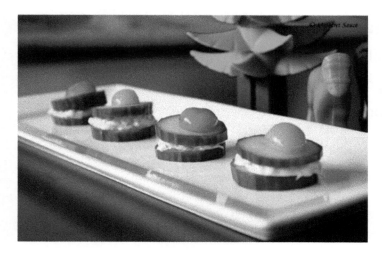

Veggie Fritters

Cooking time: 10 minutes

Servings: 4

Ingredients:

- 2 garlic cloves; minced
- 2 yellow onions; chopped
- 4 scallions; chopped
- 2 carrots; grated
- 2 teaspoons of cumin; ground
- ½ teaspoon of turmeric powder
- Salt and black pepper to the taste
- ¼ teaspoon of coriander; ground
- 2 tablespoons of parsley; chopped
- ¼ teaspoon of lemon juice
- ½ cup of almond flour
- 2 beets; peeled and grated
- 2 eggs; whisked
- ¼ cup of tapioca flour
- 3 tablespoons of olive oil

Directions:

1. In a bowl, combine the garlic with the onions, scallions, and the rest of the Ingredients except the oil. Stir well and shape medium fritters out of this mix.
2. Heat up a pan with the oil over medium-high heat, add the fritters, cook for 5 minutes on all sides, arrange on a platter and serve.

Nutrition:

1. Calories: 209
2. Fat: 11.2 g
3. Fiber: 3 g
4. Carbs: 4.4 g
5. Protein: 4.8 g

Olives and Cheese Stuffed Tomatoes

Preparation time: 10 minutes

Cooking time: 0 minutes

Servings: 24

Ingredients:

- 24 cherry tomatoes; top cut off and insides scooped out
- 2 tablespoons of olive oil
- ¼ teaspoon of red pepper flakes
- ½ cup of feta cheese; crumbled
- 2 tablespoons of black olive paste
- ¼ cup of mint; torn

Directions:

1. In a bowl, mix the olives paste with the rest of the Ingredients except the cherry tomatoes, and whisk well.
2. Stuff the cherry tomatoes with this mix, arrange them all on a platter and serve as an appetizer.

Nutrition:

- Calories: 136
- Fat: 8.6 g
- Fiber: 4.8 g
- Carbs: 5.6 g
- Protein: 5.1 g

Cucumber Sandwich Bites

Preparation time: 5 minutes

Cooking time: 0 minutes

Servings: 12

Ingredients:

- 1 cucumber; sliced
- 8 slices of whole wheat bread
- 2 tablespoons of cream cheese; soft
- 1 tablespoon of chives; chopped
- ¼ cup of avocado; peeled, pitted and mashed
- 1 teaspoon of mustard
- Salt and black pepper to the taste

Directions:

1. Spread the mashed avocado on each bread slice, also spread the rest of the Ingredients except the cucumber slices.
2. Divide the cucumber slices on the bread slices, cut each slice in thirds, arrange on a platter and serve as an appetizer.

Nutrition:

- Calories: 187
- Fat: 12.4 g
- Fiber: 2.1 g
- Carbs: 4.5 g
- Protein 8.2 g

White Bean Dip

Cooking time: 0 minute

Servings: 4

Ingredients:

- 15 ounces of canned white beans; drained and rinsed
- 6 ounces of canned artichoke hearts; drained and quartered
- 4 garlic cloves; minced
- 1 tablespoon of basil; chopped
- 2 tablespoons of olive oil
- Juice of ½ lemon
- Zest of ½ lemon; grated
- Salt and black pepper to the taste

Directions:

1. In your food processor, mix the beans with the artichokes and the rest of the Ingredients except the oil and pulse well.
2. Add the oil gradually, pulse the combination again, divide into cups and serve with a celebration dip.

Nutrition:

- Calories: 274
- Fat: 11.7 g
- Fiber: 6.5 g
- Carbs: 18.5 g
- Protein: 16.5 g

Eggplant Dip

Cooking time: 40 minutes

Servings: 4

Ingredients:

- 1 eggplant; poked with a fork
- 2 tablespoons of tahini paste
- 2 tablespoons of lemon juice
- 2 garlic cloves; minced
- 1 tablespoon of olive oil
- Salt and black pepper to the taste
- 1 tablespoon of parsley; chopped

Directions:

1. Put the eggplant in a roasting pan, bake at 400°F for 40 minutes, allow to cool down, then peel and transfer to your food processor.
2. Add the rest of the Ingredients except the parsley, pulse well, divide into small bowls and serve an appetizer with the parsley sprinkled on top.

Nutrition:

- Calories: 121
- Fat: 4.3 g
- Fiber: 1 g
- Carbs: 1.4 g
- Protein: 4.3 g

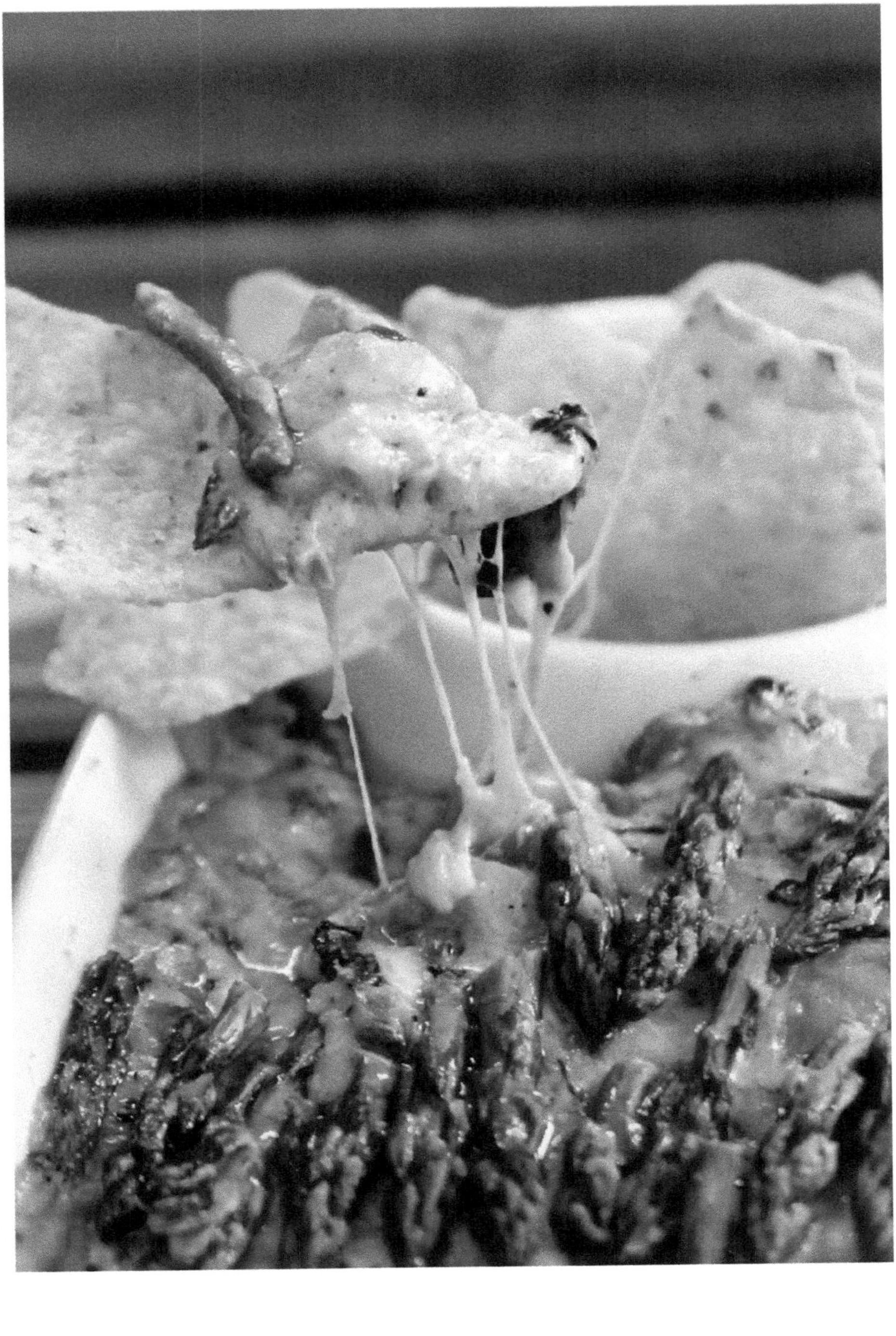

Lightning Source UK Ltd.
Milton Keynes UK
UKHW020807180621
385732UK00001B/85